P...
Rotherham Prim
Oak House
Moorhead Way
Bramley
Rotherham S66 1YY
Tel. No. 01709 302096

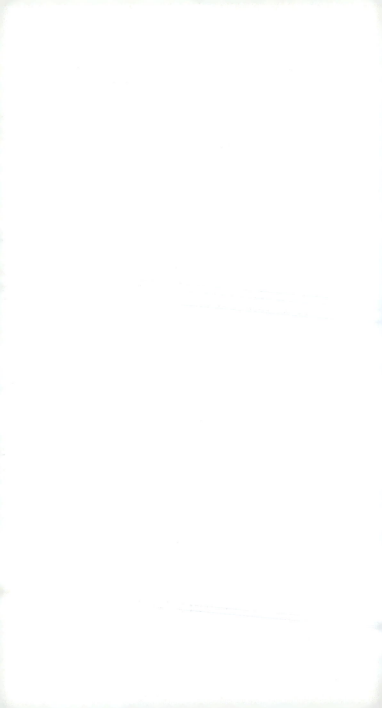

Nails
Appearance and Therapy

Second Edition

David de Berker
Bristol Dermatology Centre, UK

Ivan Bristow
*Podiatrist, University College
Northampton, UK*

Robert Baran
Nail Disease Centre, Cannes, France

Rodney PR Dawber
*Oxford Hair Foundation
Churchill Hospital, Oxford, UK*

MARTIN DUNITZ

© 1993, 2002, Martin Dunitz Ltd, a member of Taylor & Francis group

First published in the United Kingdom in 1993
by Martin Dunitz Ltd, The Livery House, 7–9 Pratt Street, London NW1 0AE

Tel: +44 (0) 20 74822202
Fax: +44 (0) 20 72670159
E-mail: info@dunitz.co.uk
Website: http://www.dunitz.co.uk

Second edition 2002

A CIP record for this book is available from the British Library

ISBN 1 84184 184 6

Distributed in the USA by
Fulfilment Center, Taylor & Francis
7625 Empire Drive, Florence, KY 41042, USA
Toll Free Tel: +1 800 634 7064
Email: cserve@routledge_ny.com

Distributed in Canada by
Taylor & Francis, 74 Rolark Drive
Scarborough, Ontario M1R 4G2, Canada
Toll Free Tel: +1 877 226 2237
Email: tal_fran@istar.ca

Distributed in the rest of the world by
Thomson Publishing Services Limited, Cheriton House, North Way, Andover
Hampshire SP10 5BE, UK
Tel: +44 (0)1264 332424
Email: salesorder.tandf@thomsonpublishingservices.co.uk

Printed and bound in Italy by Printer Trento S.r.l.

Contents

Section One: Physical signs

Section Two: Diseases and their treatment

Introduction

This book is oriented towards the most practical of practitioners. It is concise, without discussion of rarities or complex therapeutic choices. The emphasis is on the recognition of signs, classification of disease and what to do next. To do nothing may sometimes be the best advice, but it needs to be given with the confidence that this book will promote.

Further reading includes:

Baran R, Dawber RPR, de Berker DAR, Haneke E, Tosti A, *Baran and Dawber's Diseases of the Nails and their Management* (Blackwell: Oxford, 3rd edn, 2001).

Baran R, Dawber RPR, Tosti A, Haneke E, *Text Atlas of Nail Disorders* (Martin Dunitz: London, 1996).

Dawber R, Bristow I, Turner W, *Text Atlas of Podiatric Dermatology* (Martin Dunitz: London, 2001).

Clubbing

Definition

The following features define clubbing.

1. Increased nail curvature

2. Hypertrophy of the soft tissue at the end of the digit

3. A soft nail base which can easily be rocked, due to hyperplasia of dermal fibrovascular tissue

4. Local cyanosis in up to 60% of cases.

Increased convexity of the nail alone is an inadequate sign on which to base the diagnosis of clubbing.

Lovibond, Curth and Schamroth have given their names to the diagnostic angles of altered curvature seen in clubbing, as illustrated in Figure 1.

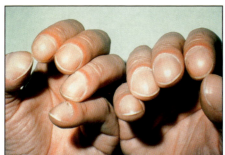

Figure 1a
Clubbing.

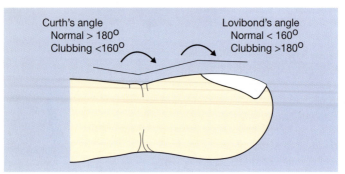

Curth's angle
Normal > 180°
Clubbing <160°

Lovibond's angle
Normal < 160°
Clubbing >180°

Figure 1b
The angles of Lovibond and Curth in nail clubbing.

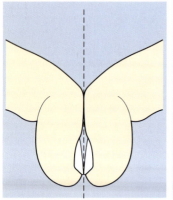

Figure 1c
Schamroth's window in normal nails.

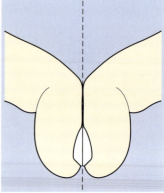

Figure 1d
Schamroth's window is lost in clubbing.

Hypertrophic pulmonary osteoarthropathy

This is a variant of clubbing associated with a thoracic neoplasm or bronchiectasis. Clubbing is a central feature, seen with:

1. Acromegalic changes of the hands and feet

2. Arthropathy of the large limb joints, especially of the legs

3. Radiological changes of bilateral proliferative periostitis

4. Peripheral neurovascular disorders, e.g. local cyanosis and parasthesia

Causes

The causes of clubbing are as follows.

Idiopathic Acquired	
Thoracic	**Bronchiectasis, fibrotic lung disease, emphysema, neoplasm**, abscess, chronic pulmonary sepsis, tuberculosis, *Pneumocystis carinii* infection
Cardiovascular	Congenital cyanotic heart disease, atrial myxoma
Alimentary (5%)	Gastrointestinal neoplasm, small and large bowel inflammation, e.g. Crohn's disease and ulcerative colitis
Endocrine	**Cirrhosis**, chronic active hepatitis, autoimmune thyroiditis
General	Polycythaemia with hypoxia, malnutrition
Limited to few digits	Brachial plexus damage, aortic or a subclavian artery aneurysm, sarcoid, gout
Lower limbs	Abdominal aortic graft with sepsis

Koilonychia

Definition

Koilonychia is a transverse and longitudinal concave nail dystrophy giving a spoon-shaped appearance (Figure 2). It is associated with any condition which causes thinning of the nail. Children's toenails may show an idiopathic form which resolves with age. Conversely, it may develop in the elderly and be irreversible.

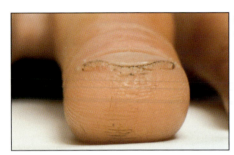

Figure 2
Koilonychia.

Causes

The causes of koilonychia are as follows.

Idiopathic	
Physiological	**Early childhood**
Congenital	Trichothiodystrophy, ectodermal dysplasias, nail–patella syndrome
Metabolic	**Iron deficiency**, haemochromatosis, porphyria, renal dialysis/transplant, thyroid disease
Dermatoses	**Lichen planus, alopecia areata**, psoriasis, Darier's disease, Raynaud's disease
Occupational	**e.g contact with oils**
Infective	Onychomycosis

Splinter haemorrhages

Definition

These are **linear haemorrhages 2–3 mm in length, usually in the longitudinal axis of the nail bed**. They are generally non-specific phenomenona, which in small numbers on a single digit are of no significance (Figure 3).

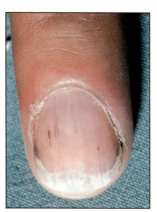

Figure 3a
Splinter haemorrhages.
Longitudinal haemorrhages seen through the nail plate.

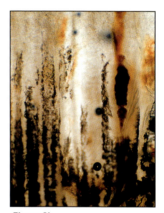

Figure 3b
Splinter haemorrhages.
Haem staining light brown on the grooved under-surface of the nail plate.

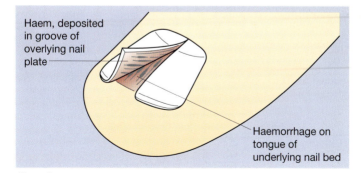

Figure 3c
Splinter haemorrhages. Mechanism of splinter haemorrhage formation.

They are most often distally located; in onychomatricoma, a matrix tumour, they are proximal.

The causes of splinter haemorrhages are as follows.

Idiopathic	
Local trauma	
Local dermatoses	**Eczema, psoriasis, onychomycosis** scurvy, pemphigus
	Collagen/vascular disease, Raynaud's disease, antiphospholipid syndrome
Vessel infarction	Septicaemia, e.g endocarditis and septic emboli
	Blood dyscrasia, hepatitis and cirrhosis
	Severe illness

Other shapes

Pincer (involution) deformity

Pincer deformity is caused by a **transverse overcurvature that increases distally**. This is cosmetically undesirable and occasionally painful (Figure 4). On the feet it has been attributed to ill-fitting shoes or distortion of the proximal nail matrix by osteophytes (see *Ingrowing nails*). Asymmetrical pincer deformity, or pincer deformity with nail discoloration and disintegration, may betray a subungual tumour. This may be a soft tissue tumour, such as a glomus (see *Non-melanoma tumours*) or a bony tumour such as a subungual exostosis which should be investigated by X-ray. Distal overcurvature may eventually produce loss of nail bed and funnel or claw formation.

Racquet thumb

Racquet thumb results from a **disproportionately broad nail bed on the thumb when the distal phalanx is**

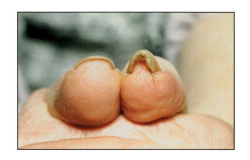

Figure 4a
Pincer nail.

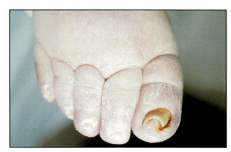

Figure 4b
Involuted (pincer) nail.

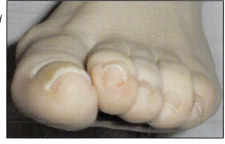

Figure 4c
Appearance of an involuted nail following conservative resection.

shorter than normal; the wider the nail, the narrower the lateral nail folds (Figure 5). This is a common, isolated, autosomally dominant condition, occasionally reported in association with other abnormalities. Psoriatic arthropathy and resorption of the terminal phalanx in hypoparathyroidism can produce the same effect. Acquired unilateral racquet thumb may be due to an underlying neoplasm.

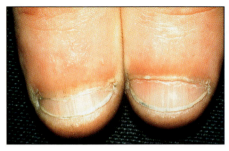
Figure 5
Racquet thumb.

Hook and claw nails

The nail as it grows adheres to the terminal aspect of the digit pulp, curving onto the plantar surface. This condition often affects the fifth toes, where there is trauma from high heels, or other toes after fracture of the terminal phalanx. It is occasionally congenital or may be associated with nail–patella syndrome.

Nail atrophy

Definition

Nail atrophy occurs when there is a reduction in surface area and thickness of the nail, often accompanied by splitting and variable loss (Figure 6). With some scarring forms of nail atrophy a pterygium (ridge of fibrous tissue) may develop. A dorsal pterygium involves a fibrotic extension of the proximal nail fold into the adjacent nail bed. A ventral pterygium is a similar process but occurs subungually and is visible distally. A dorsal pterygium will always result in some permanent disfigurement.

Figure 6a
Lichen planus nail atrophy.

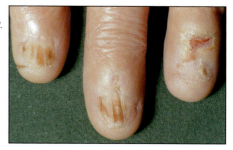

Figure 6b
Psoriatic nail atrophy.

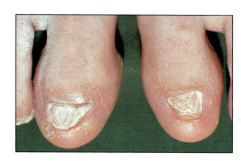

Causes

The causes of nail atrophy are as follows.

Atrophy with potential for pterygium	Lichen planus, acrosclerosis
	Onychotillomania, Lesch–Nyhan syndrome, chronic graft rejection
	Stevens–Johnson or Lyell's syndrome
	Cicatricial pemphigoid
Atrophy with no pterygium potential	**Severe paronychia with dystrophy**
	Idiopathic atrophy of childhood
	Severe psoriatic nail disease
	Epidermolysis bullosa
	Amyloid and retinoid nail dystrophy

Pitting

Definition

Pits are small erosions in the nail surface. It is arbitrary to provide a number that can be accepted as not pathological, but to find a total of five in the otherwise normal nails of both hands is common. Pits may help in the diagnosis of psoriasis, especially when they are deep and irregularly shaped, but they are not pathognomonic of any disease (Figure 7).

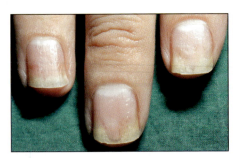

Figure 7a
Psoriatic pits.

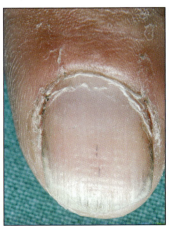

Figure 7b
Alopecia areata pits.

Causes

The causes of pitting are as follows.

Psoriasis

Alopecia areata

Eczema

Occupational trauma

Parakeratosis pustulosa

Pityriasis rosea, secondary syphilis, sarcoid, lichen planus, Reiters' syndrome

Rough nails – trachyonychia

Definition

There is a roughness of the nail surface as if it had been longitudinally rubbed with sandpaper (Figure 8). In more extreme forms the nail becomes brittle and fragments at the free edge.

Figure 8
Trachyonychia.

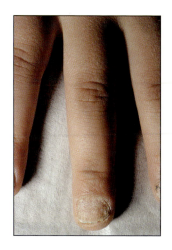

Causes

There are several causes of trachyonychia, the most common being an idiopathic '20-nail dystrophy' (which may not always involve all 20 nails). This has a variable association with autoimmune disorders, particularly lichen planus and alopecia areata. Complete or partial resolution is likely in children, but not in adults.

Idiopathic 20-nail dystrophy

Alopecia areata

Lichen planus

Chemicals

Ichthyosis vulgaris, ectodermal dysplasia, selective IgA deficiency, systemic amyloid

---

Nail splitting – onychoschizia

Definition

Nail splitting that involves the proximal nail is longitudinal throughout the nail, and is of matrix origin. Distal splitting

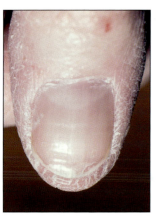

Figure 9
Terminal onychoschizia.

into layers is usually transverse, and most commonly results from weathering (Figure 9).

Causes

The causes of nail splitting are as follows.

Proximal	Psoriasis
	Lichen planus
	Retinoid therapy
	Tumours beneath the nail matrix, e.g. glomus, myxoid cyst
Distal	Repeated wetting
	Old age
	Chemical damage
	Polycythaemia rubra vera

Onycholysis

Definition

Onycholysis is a separation of the nail from the nail bed at the distal or lateral margins (Figure 10). The split is made apparent by a change in the normal pink colour seen through the nail. Pus, air and shed squames give a yellow appearance. Pseudomonas imparts a green hue, and blood appears red-brown or black. Serum-like exudate containing glycoproteins produces an 'oily spot' or 'salmon patch' as seen in psoriasis.

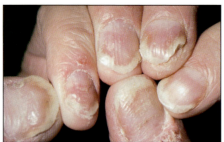

Figure 10a
Psoriatic onycholysis.

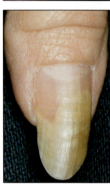

Figure 10b
Fungal onycholysis due to Candida sp.

Causes

By far the most common causes of onycholysis are fungus/candida, psoriasis and trauma, as follows.

Psoriasis	
Infection	**Fungus/candida**, bacteria, warts, subungual corns
Trauma	**Especially shoes and manicure**
Eczema	**Contact and endogenous**
Chemicals	**Paint remover and other solvents**
Dermatoses	Lichen planus, blistering disorders, Reiter's disease
Systemic	Tumours, peripheral vascular disease, collagen vascular disease
Photosensitivity (rarely in toes)	Thiazide, psoralen, tetracycline, doxycycline

Nail loss – onychomadesis

Definition

Onychomadesis is the complete loss of all or a large part of a nail due to a split developing in the proximal part of the nail unit (Figure 11).

Figure 11
Bullous onychomadesis.

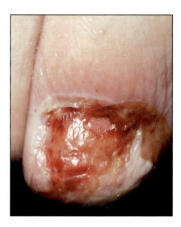

Causes

Nails may be shed for any of the reasons that onycholysis develops, representing an extreme of this phenomenon. In addition there are causes that focus on the matrix, as follows.

Local inflammation, e.g. acute paronychia

Local trauma

Fever/systemic upset

Bullous dermatoses, e.g. pemphigus

Stevens–Johnson syndrome and toxic epidermal necrolysis

Drugs: cytotoxics, antibiotics, retinoids

Kawasaki syndrome

Thick nails – pachyonychia / onychauxis

Definition

A normal fingernail is about 0.5 mm thick and a toenail twice this. **Hyperkeratosis of the nail bed may cause apparent thickening, whereas changes in the matrix result in real thickening** (Figure 12). Often the two occur together. Typically the nail assumes a yellow-brown discoloration. In the foot, the acquired thickening is seen often in the first and fifth toenails as a result of damage from ill-fitting footwear or a single trauma to the nail. Hypertrophy of the nail plate makes nail-cutting difficult, and subsequent pressure on the nail from footwear may cause pain. Secondary fungal infection may follow (see *Onychomycosis*). **Onychogryphosis** is a thickened nail which is long, due to lack of cutting, and distorted, due to footwear and/or hallux valgus. Onychogryphosis usually involves the great toe of the elderly, and is occasionally related to vascular abnormalities in the affected limb.

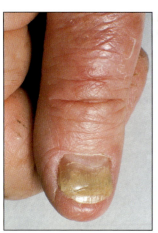

Figure 12a
Psoriatic thickening.

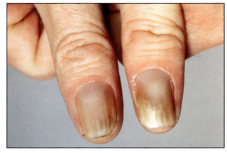

Figure 12b
Pachyonychia congenita.

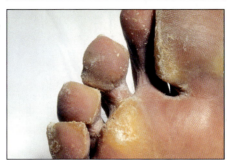

Figure 12c
Associated palmar–plantar hyperkeratosis.

Causes

Causes of thick nails are as follows.

Real thickening (matrix)	**Psoriasis/Reiter's disease**
	Onychomycosis
	Trauma
	Contact eczema
	Lichen planus
	Alopecia areata
Apparent thickening	**Onychomycosis**
	Chronic eczema
	Lichen planus
	Psoriasis

Grooves – longitudinal

Definition

A longitudinal groove is straight and usually arises from beneath the proximal nail fold (Figure 13). The groove may be singular (often wide) or multiple and of variable width.

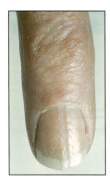

Figure 13
Longitudinal grooves – any cause.

Causes

The causes of longitudinal grooves are as follows.

Multiple grooves	Normal, increasing with age
	Associated with atrophic nails (see *Nail atrophy*)
	Vascular insufficiency, e.g. collagen vascular disease, rheumatoid arthritis
	Peripheral vascular disease, frostbite
Single grooves	Familial
	Trauma
	Tumours, e.g pseudomyxoid cyst, fibroma
	Median canaliform dystrophy

Chromonychia

Abnormalities of colour depend on the transparency of the nail, its attachments and the character of the underlying tissue. If the causes are exogenous, such as occupational exposure or topical medication, the discoloration tends to follow the contour of the proximal nail fold. With endogenous causes, the changes correspond to the shape of the lunula (Figure 14).

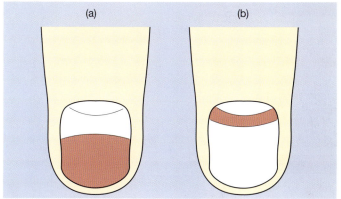

Figure 14
The distinction between (a) exogenous and (b) endogenous chromonychia.

Leuconychia

Definition

In **true leuconychia** the abnormality originates in the matrix and the nail appears white. It may take any of four forms: affecting the entire nail, as longitudinal or as transverse lines, or as isolated white patches (Figure 15).

Pseudoleuconychia is a white nail caused by disease outside the matrix, e.g. onychomycosis (Figure 16).

Figure 15
True leuconychia.

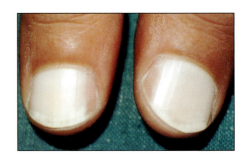

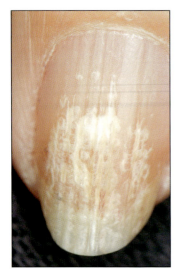

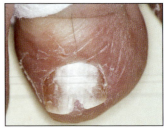

Figure 16a (above)
Pseudoleuconychia due to superficial aspergillus infection.

Figure 16b (left)
Pseudoleuconychia due to nail varnish.

Apparent leuconychia is a spurious whiteness due to changes in subungual tissues (Figure 17).

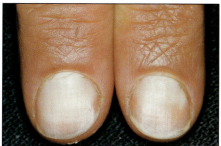

Figure 17a
Apparent leuconychia with renal failure.

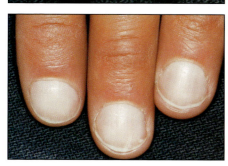

Figure 17b
Apparent leuconychia with hypoalbuminaemia.

Causes

The causes of leuconychia are as follows.

True leuconychia	**Psoriasis**
	Exfoliative dermatitis
	Trauma
	Alopecia areata, gout, heavy-metal poisoning, shock, renal failure, zinc deficiency
Pseudoleuconychia	**Onychomycosis**
	Nail varnish
Apparent leuconychia	**Anaemia**
	Hypoalbuminaemia
	Renal disease
	Onycholysis

Melanonychia

Definition

Melanonychia is a black or brown discoloration of the nail, usually localised and often longitudinal (Figure 18).

Biological melanonychia is due to either haem or melanin on the under surface of the nail or in the nail itself. Artefactual melanonychia is produced by exogenous pigment, such as tobacco, potassium permanganate or henna on the outer surface. Clinically, the critical decision is whether the pigment derives from a malignant melanoma.

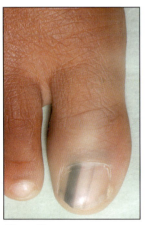

Figure 18a
Racial melanonychia.

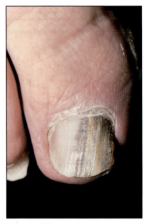

Figure 18b
Onychomycosis melanonychia.

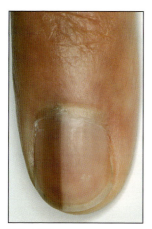

Figure 18c
Longitudinal melanonychia with Hutchinson's sign on proximal nail fold.

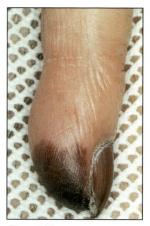

Figure 18d
Melanoma of the nail unit extending onto the finger pulp.

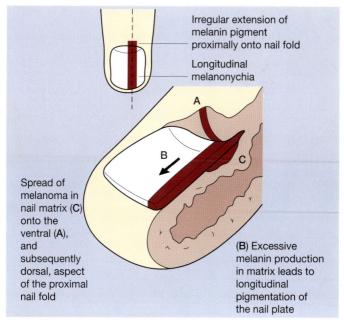

Irregular extension of melanin pigment proximally onto nail fold

Longitudinal melanonychia

A

B

C

Spread of melanoma in nail matrix (C) onto the ventral (A), and subsequently dorsal, aspect of the proximal nail fold

(B) Excessive melanin production in matrix leads to longitudinal pigmentation of the nail plate

Figure 18e
Origin of pigment in malignant melanoma of the nail unit.

Causes

The causes of melanonychia are as follows.

Biological	Idiopathic
	Racial (almost 100% of middle-aged Afro-Caribbeans)
	Trauma
	Onychomycosis
	Malignant melanoma
	Bacterial infection
	Benign melanocytic lesion, hypoadrenalism
	Laugier–Hunziker–Baran syndrome (with buccal pigmentation)
	Lichen planus
Artefactual	**Exogenous pigments**

Diagnosis

It is often necessary to make the distinction between a melanocytic lesion and a haematoma. No practitioner can be criticised for referring any melanonychia, because morbidity with subungual melanoma is high even with early diagnosis.

The first observation should be the **site of origin of the pigment**. Melanomas have only been identified arising from the matrix (i.e. from the lunula or more proximally). Haematomas may develop anywhere.

A history of trauma does not help unless it is very definite. The most valuable difference in the history is that a haematoma will grow out with the nail, unlike a melanoma.

The situation is less clear if the digit (most commonly a toe) is subject to repeated trauma, so that new haematoma is constantly produced and masks the growing-out appearance. Equally, the diagnosis is made more difficult if the haematoma is only partly attributable to trauma and there is an underlying pathology that bleeds easily. Consequently, a borehole in the nail that identifies blood is not sufficient to exclude a neoplasm. A persistent melanonychia that fails to grow out requires an expert opinion, which will usually lead to biopsy. Additional factors that make a melanoma more likely are:

- only one digit involved

- spread of the pigment onto the proximal nail fold

- rapidly (months) progressive widening, with blurred borders

- age over 50 years

- darkening of the streak.

Other nail discolorations – chromonychias

The causes of other nail discolorations are as follows.

Yellow	Onychomycosis
	Nail enamel and hardeners
	Carotene
	Drugs: mepacrine
	Jaundice
Blue/grey	Drugs: antimalarials, minocycline, phenothiazines
	Argyria

Green	*Pseudomonas aeruginosa*
	Bullous disorders
	Ageing haematoma
Red/purple	Glomus tumour
	Warfarin
	Angioma
	Enchondroma
	Darier's disease
	Lupus erythematosus
Brown	Malnutrition
	Nail cosmetics
	Thyroid disease
	Pregnancy
	Dithranol, potassium permanganate, silver nitrate, *Proteus mirabilis, Candida albicans*

Treatment

Most nail diseases involve disruption of the hard nail structure and its smooth resistant surface. Consequently, part of any therapy involves protection of the nail and periungual region from damaging substances, irritants and trauma.

This may mean wearing gloves at work and during wet work at home. There should be routine avoidance of grease-cutting agents, such as soap and detergent. An emollient should be used as a soap substitute and moisturiser. These measures are fundamental to the care of a dystrophic nail and should be part of all therapies.

With the toenails, avoidance of physical trauma is an important aspect of therapy. In most cases this is a result of occupational hazards, foot shape and footwear. It is therefore essential to anticipate these issues to avoid problems. The common problems with footwear are summarised below. Where the foot position (e.g. hallux valgus, flat foot, digital deformity) predisposes to nail problems, orthotic therapy with in-shoe devices may help to redistribute foot pressures, realign toes and relieve trauma to the nails.

Problem	Effect
Unsuitable fastening	Foot moves forward in shoe, traumatising nail unit. If shoe is loose, toes will claw to maintain stability, further compromising nail structure
Excessive heel height	Foot forced forward into shoe as above
Inadequate toe box depth or width	Compression of toes
Occlusive construction	Increases in-shoe temperature, sweating and microbial growth

Onychomycosis

Definition

Onychomycosis is a **fungal infection of the nail apparatus** (Figure 19). This may involve the nail bed, matrix and plate, either in isolation or together. The main pathogen is *Trichophyton* sp., but *Scopularopsis brevicaulis* is sometimes isolated, typically when there is a cloudy infection of half the nail of one great toe. Yeasts (*Candida albicans*) and pseudomonas infections may occur alone or in association with a fungus. Pseudomonas infections give rise to a characteristic green colour.

The terminology of the location of a fungal infection is described in Figure 19a.

Diagnosis
Nail clippings and subungual scrapings
Part of the sample can be examined under the microscope in the surgery after soaking in 20 to 30% potassium hydroxide solution to dissolve the keratin. The rest should be sent for mycology. Specimens survive well in the post, and the accuracy of the result is increased if the nail

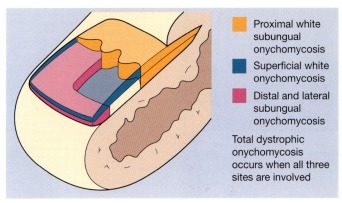

Proximal white subungual onychomycosis

Superficial white onychomycosis

Distal and lateral subungual onychomycosis

Total dystrophic onychomycosis occurs when all three sites are involved

Figure 19a
The different patterns of onychomycosis.

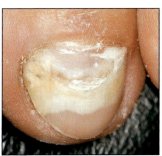

Figure 19b
Proximal onychomycosis.

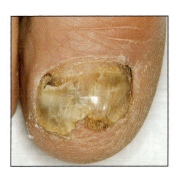

Figure 19c
Distal and lateral onychomycosis due to Trichophyton rubrum.

Figure 19d
Total dystrophic onychomycosis due to a saprophyte infection.

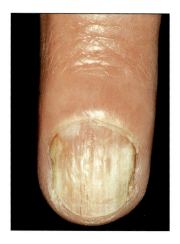

Figure 19e
Candidal nail plate infection.

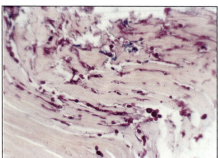

Figure 19f
Fungal nail histology.

sample exceeds 3 mm in width. Crumbly matter from under the nail is a good source of infected material, and as much as possible should be included in the sample.

Nail biopsy

This is not routinely recommended. However, the pathological identification of fungi does require periodic acid-Schiff (PAS) staining of an isolated sample of nail and associated subungual material. A substantial specimen of nail and underlying tissue is needed, such as a 3 to 4 mm punch biopsy.

It is important to recognise that the isolation of fungus from a dystrophic nail does not prove that this is the cause of the dystrophy. An established dystrophy is susceptible to colonisation by fungus, which may further damage the nail. This can sometimes account for the lack of complete resolution of a presumed onychomycosis after appropriate treatment. Equally, the presence of a fungus is not fully excluded by negative microbiology, as a trial of therapy may show in some cases.

A biopsy is most helpful if the differential diagnosis of psoriasis or another dermatosis is being considered; in such cases the nail and underlying tissue should be biopsied. This procedure may cause scarring, and is best performed by a practitioner familiar with the technique.

Treatment
Topical
Amorolfine (Loceryl®), applied once weekly, and 8% ciclopiroxolamine, applied daily, are nail lacquers which act as transungual delivery systems. They are most effective when the lunula is spared. Trosyl® (28% tioconazole solution) is of limited value. The other topical antifungals are best used in conjunction with urea avulsion (see *Surgical* systemic treatment). Where nails are thickened, penetration by topical preparations may be enhanced by reducing the thickness with a nail drill.

Systemic
Terbinafine is licensed for use in a 6-week course for the treatment of fingernail onychomycosis, and for a 12-week course for toenails at a dose of 250 mg daily. Shorter courses of treatment can still be effective; this probably reflects the fungicidal character of the drug. Fungistatic drugs often require more prolonged courses of treatment. Trials suggest that the cure rate is 50–80%, with a modest relapse rate in the first year. Success is more likely if the

fungus is one of the more common types known as a der-matophyte, and if the infected nail plate is not too bulky. The drug has relatively few side-effects, the most frequent-ly reported complaint being temporary loss of taste. It is not clear how long the drug remains in fat nor how this affects advice to women who may subsequently want to become pregnant. The current recommendation is that conception within 6 months of the last dose should be avoided.

Itraconazole, which may give similar results, is advocated as a pulse therapy. Each pulse comprises a 1-week course of 200 mg itraconazole twice daily. Fingernail treatment requires 2 pulses over 2 months (i.e. in weeks 1 and 5) and toenails require 3 pulses over 3 months (i.e. in weeks 1, 5 and 9). Itraconazole is effective against *Candida*, whereas terbinafine is barely so, but it exhibits more drug interactions than terbinafine. It is important that concurrent and incidental medications such as antibiotics and antihist-amines be checked against the drug information sheet before prescribing.

Griseofulvin has the advantage of being cheap and of known safety in long courses and in children. It has, however, a higher incidence of side-effects such as gas-trointestinal upset and rashes. A 6-month course of griseofulvin is required for fingernails and a 12- to 18-month course for toenails; the ideal duration is 1 month longer in each case, to ensure clinical clearance. In patients with frequent relapses, it has also been suggested that the prophylactic use of an antifungal nail lacquer might keep the nails disease-free. Griseofulvin is of no use in *Candida* infections.

Combined therapy
There is an argument for combining topical and systemic therapies, if experience has shown that monotherapy in a

particular patient is ineffective. Recent data suggest that a combination of, for example, amorolfine with terbinafine may yield a higher cure rate for dermatophyte nail infections involving the matrix.

Surgical

Complete surgical avulsion is not usually recommended: bacterial wound infection and distal ingrowing are potential postoperative complications. These problems are often avoided by removal of only part of the nail, or by chemical avulsion using 40% urea paste applied daily under a dressing. This causes keratinolysis and hence disintegration of diseased nail over 2 to 6 weeks. The softened nail can easily be pared away, which increases the efficacy of both topical and systemic antifungal treatment.

Prognosis

Relapse is common, and therefore measures should be taken to reduce the risk of re-infection. In pedal onychomycosis, footwear should have suitable fastening, a low heel and adequate space in the toe box, in order to avoid further nail trauma. Onychomycosis frequently occurs secondary to other skin infection, and so careful foot hygiene with the regular application of topical antifungal creams should be encouraged. Antifungal powders dusted into footwear are also of benefit.

Psoriasis

Definition

The ungual features of psoriasis include pitting, thickening, onycholysis, discoloration, oily spots, paronychia and splinter haemorrhages (Figure 20).

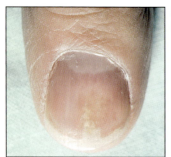

Figure 20a
Oily spots and pits in psoriasis.

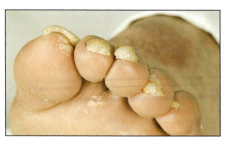

Figure 20b
Subungual hyperkeratosis in psoriasis.

Treatment

In some patients, improvement in the general condition may be matched by improvement in the nails. Keeping the nails short and avoiding manicure minimises the isomorphic response in the nail unit; trauma can provoke psoriasis. General hand and foot care with emollient and protective measures to avoid trauma are advisable. Systemic or topical lacquer antifungals may inadvertently help if onychomycosis and nail psoriasis coexist.

Topical

Topical medication can reduce onycholysis, thickening and periungual scale.

After emollient, the most common topical therapy is steroid. A potent or very potent steroid may need to be applied to the proximal nail fold or to the free edge over 2 to 3 months. Access is limited, but it is possible to clip the nail right back to the transverse level of the split and to treat with steroid ointment as the nail regrows. Isolated fingernail involvement may benefit from intralesional triamcinolone (2.5 mg/ml) injected into the proximal nail fold, when the disease affects the matrix.

Long-term use of a strong steroid can result in atrophy of the periungual soft tissues and therefore cannot be maintained indefinitely. Calcipotriol is an alternative where the main problem is subungual hyperkeratosis, and this is safe long term.

Distal disease of an isolated fingernail can be treated with injections of the hyponychium with steroid and local anaesthetic (there must be **no adrenaline** in the lignocaine). Prolonged therapy should be balanced against local atrophy.

Liquid antipsoriatic scalp applications may be used to treat the nail bed if onycholysis is a feature.

Hospital therapy
Acitretin is most helpful for the very thick nails found in some psoriatics. The benefits are usually seen when the treatment is indicated for widespread psoriasis of the skin. Acropustulosis continua is a distinct form of pustular psoriasis found in isolated digits: this may be an indication for the use of retinoids. Pitting and onycholysis can be made worse by retinoids.

Psoralen UVA (PUVA) may help as both general and local treatment. If applied locally alone it results in odd discoloration due to tanning. Its use requires high doses of UVA, with the risk of photoonycholysis. It is rarely effective in the toenails because the nail plate is too thick to allow penetration of sufficient UVA. However, a systemic benefit from whole-body PUVA may be seen in the toenails several months after completion of the course of therapy.

Methotrexate and cyclosporin improve ungual psoriasis as part of generalised psoriasis treatment.

Surgical

Surgical treatment may be an option where there is significant nail-plate distortion with upgrowing or ingrowing, especially in the toenails.

Prognosis

Specific treatments may help during periods of exacerbation. General measures are of some benefit and should be used at all times. Nail disease affects only 7% of child psoriatics and becomes more prominent with age.

Microbial paronychia

Definition

Microbial paronychia is an **infective inflammatory condition of the periungual soft tissue**, usually secondary to trauma or primary dermatosis. The pattern may be of acute or chronic infection (Figure 21).

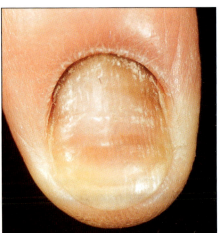

Figure 21a
Chronic paronychia.

Figure 21b
Vasculitic paronychia.

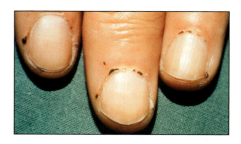

Figure 21c
Eczematous paronychia.

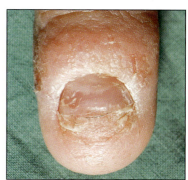

Causes

The causes of microbial paronychia are as follows.

Predisposing	Hangnail (torn skin at edge of nail)	
	Acute trauma	
	Generalised/chronic trauma: shoes, manicure, ingrowing	
	Chronic irritation: domestic/occupational wetting, sucking	
Microbial	**Acute**	***Staphylococcus aureus***
		Streptococcus pyogenes
		Herpes simplex
	Chronic	***Trichophyton* sp.**
		***Candida* sp.**

Acute paronychia
Diagnosis

There is localised erythema and swelling of the paronychium in one digit. The history may provide evidence of trauma or aggressive manicure. The swelling may come to a head and provide pus for microbiology when incised. Alternatively, pus may be expressed from the nail fold.

Treatment

Treatment involves flucloxacillin, 500 mg four times daily (or as directed by microbiology), with chlorhexidine as a local antiseptic. If pain and swelling fail to subside within 48 hours, surgery may be needed. The focus of infection may be visible within a nail fold or may be beneath the nail, when pus is seen under the nail. In this latter location, the matrix is vulnerable to irreversible damage and failed medical treatment may require the next step of surgical drainage. Either the proximal or distal half of the nail should be removed, whichever half overlies the area of maximum tenderness. Distal removal may only require the excision of a U-shaped piece of nail.

Prognosis

This is a treatable condition with a good prognosis. The main problem is damage to the matrix with scarring if pus is not drained at an early stage; this is particularly the case with children.

Chronic paronychia
Diagnosis

The condition most commonly affects the index and middle fingers of the dominant hand. There is periungual erythema and swelling that forms a cushion at the nail fold. The adherence of the cuticle is lost and there is retraction of the proximal nail fold. This prolongs the condition, as foreign bodies and microbes become lodged beneath the nail fold causing inflammation and infection. It is sometimes possible to express pus from the nail fold. A nail dystrophy may develop secondary to the paronychia.

Certain dermatoses or systemic conditions may mimic or precipitate a chronic paronychia, as follows.

Dermatoses	Eczema (especially fresh food handlers)
	Psoriasis, Reiter's disease
	Lichen planus
	Bowen's disease, invasive squamous cell carcinoma
Systemic	Vasculitis
	Stevens–Johnson syndrome
	Neuropathy
	Metastases

Treatment

It is critical to correct predisposing factors as well as to treat infection. Occupational, domestic and personal habits need to be examined and modified. The most common reversible factor is the use of irritants such as soap and cleaning agents without adequate hand protection. These agents provoke a low-grade eczema which is then prone to secondary infection with bacteria and *Candida*. Both therapy and prevention rely greatly on keeping the hands dry. This may involve wearing cotton gloves beneath rubber when undertaking wet work. Emollient is a further element of hand care, providing some protection from solvents such as soap and water while also addressing the dryness and scale often found in chronic paronychia.

The diligent use of topical steroids is an important feature of local therapy. In adults very potent steroids may be necessary, often initially in combination with an antimicrobial that may include treatment for *Candida*. In some instances oral therapy for *Candida* may be required; intralesional steroid injections may be an option where infection is not a significant factor.

Prognosis

If an isolated predisposing factor can be identified and corrected, the prognosis is good. Most commonly the problem is multifactorial and may be based upon a chronic dermatosis such as eczema or psoriasis. In these cases constant encouragement to maintain good protective habits is needed, and rapid intervention at signs of relapse.

Periungual and subungual warts

Definition

Human papillomavirus infection of the periungual skin and nail apparatus causes periungual and subungual warts (Figure 22).

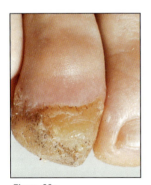

Figure 22a
Varieties of periungual warts: nail thickening.

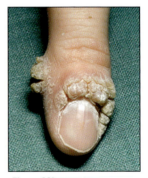

Figure 22b
Varieties of periungual warts: renal transplant patient.

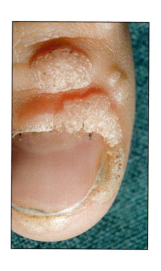

Figure 22c
Varieties of periungual warts: finger-biting.

Diagnosis

The diagnosis is usually obvious from the appearance and association with warts elsewhere. Paring the surface may give the characteristic pinpoint bleeding seen in all vital warts.

Warts beneath the nail should be exposed for assessment. They may reflect an underlying bony exostosis which can be revealed by X-ray (plane and lateral). Longstanding atypical warts in adults occasionally turn out to be squamous cell carcinoma and therefore warrant biopsy.

Treatment

The warts will go without treatment, although ungual and plantar warts can persist longer than those at other sites. This may reflect the isomorphic response where trauma provokes a continuation of the disease.

Salicylic acid

This treatment is often unsuccessful and can be messy. Great emphasis must be laid upon the correct use of the preparations; these are of up to 50% salicylic acid in an ointment base, or 17% as a collodion. It is essential that the patient soak and abrade the wart daily before reapplication. Success may be maximised by asking the patient to commence treatment under the supervision of the practice nurse.

Liquid nitrogen

This is painful and should rarely be used in children. There is little published evidence to suggest that it is more effective than properly applied salicylic acid. There is the potential for scarring the matrix with aggressive freezing. To minimise this, some practitioners use an oblique jet from the gun rather than directing it straight down upon the wart. One or two 5-second freezes are advised. Often the dose will increase on subsequent visits, but rarely exceeds two 10-second freezes on a periungual wart. It is important to use judgement to avoid the distress caused by over-treatment. Pain and erythema may be reduced by a single application of very potent steroid. The treatment should be repeated at 3 weeks and, if the patient is able to use salicylic acid preparations in the meantime, the success rate may be higher.

Bleomycin

This therapy is occasionally used in hospitals; it should not be used in general practice. Bleomycin is a cytotoxic drug which is painful when injected directly into the wart. If used around the matrix, scarring nail dystrophy may result. It is reserved for particularly troublesome warts, usually in immunosuppressed patients. Its use carries the risk of long-term Raynaud's disease as a complication.

Surgery

As a rule, this should be avoided: there is a risk of scarring at the proximal nail fold. Subungual or lateral nailfold warts may respond successfully to curettage, but it should be performed with care.

Other agents

There are many other agents used in the treatment of warts, but none of these is commonly or reliably used in the UK. The most common are as follows.

Agent	Mode of action
Cantharidin	Topical beetle extract causes epithelial cells to disintegrate
Imiquimod	Immunomodulator enhances T cell activity. Used topically in genital warts, and in combined therapy of digital warts
Laser	CO_2 laser can be used as a destructive agent
Diphencyprone	Patients are sensitised to this substance, which is then applied to provoke an allergic response with the wart as the epicentre.
Trichloracetic acid, phenol, monochloracetic + 40% salicylic acid plaster	All can be used as destructive caustic agents, normally with a local anaesthetic.

Prognosis

Warts go away, although this may take years in adults. Therapy is the more successful as it becomes more aggressive, but it is important to use judgement and to approach the problem of warts and patient as a whole. Warts also come back, particularly in nail-biters!

Lichen planus

Definition

Lichen planus characteristically affects the skin of both adults and children, in the form of **flat-topped violaceous papules with white (Wickham's) striae on mucosal**

surfaces. It can affect the scalp and axillae, to produce a scarring alopecia, and also affects the nails (Figure 23).

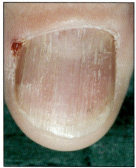

Figure 23a
Trachyonychia/lichen planus.

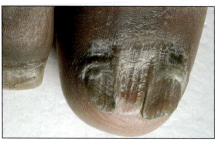

Figure 23b
Fibrotic lichen planus with pterygium.

Diagnosis

The nail changes cover a wide range of appearances and occur in 10% of those with skin involvement. In this 10% the diagnosis is relatively easy. Otherwise, diagnosis is based upon clinical judgement or histology of a longitudinal nail biopsy. Biopsy should be carried out early by a skilled operator, or the characteristic features of lichen planus may be replaced by scar tissue.

The mildest, non-specific features of lichen planus consist of longitudinal ridges or depressions in the nails and occasionally pitting. A more global atrophy of the nail matrix may produce nail fragility and a sandpaper appearance, sometimes with koilonychia. This can affect a few or all of the nails. More aggressive still is the atrophy that combines with scarring of the matrix and proximal nail fold. This results in pterygium formation, where the nail may split longitudinally and be partly or completely lost, leaving a fibrotic, atrophic nail bed.

Treatment

This varies with the type of dystrophy and is generally of limited success.

No treatment

The sandpaper dystrophy in children is best left alone; prolonged use of potent topical steroids may fuse the underlying epiphysis. If the condition is asymptomatic with scarring dystrophy and is not progressing, the scarring will not be reversed by therapy.

Steroids

Symptomatic and progressive lichen planus is treated with steroids, with mandatory histology beforehand. Oral rethoids are an alternative. Steroids can be used in several ways:

- Potent topical steroid may be massaged into the digit from the distal interphalangeal crease distally, including underneath the proximal nail fold. This should be tried for 3 months, with baseline photography for comparison.

- Injection into the proximal nail fold of 0.5 ml triamcinolone acetonide (40 mg/ml) with 0.25 ml 1% lignocaine can be carried out on several digits monthly for 6 months, and then at 2 to 6 monthly intervals. The treatment is unpleasant, and cumulatively it may constitute a large systemic dose of steroid. A more intermittent regimen with smaller doses of steroid may give some success. All the usual contraindications to systemic steroids should be considered.

- Prednisolone, 60 mg daily for the initial 4 to 6 weeks, has been advocated in extreme cases. It should then be tailed off over the next year. It may only provide temporary cosmetic relief, with considerable systemic side-effects.

- Retinoids (acitretin) can work well but side-effects may limit their use.

Prognosis

Childhood sandpaper nails have a good prognosis. Less severe forms of dystrophy coinciding with transient cutaneous lichen planus also have a good prognosis.

A dystrophy with a pterygium has scarred the matrix, and there will never be a full recovery at whatever age of onset or treatment. Adult sandpaper nails are less likely than the childhood form to resolve spontaneously.

Eczema

Definition

Eczema covers a **broad category of dermatoses with certain histological features in common: spongiosis, acanthosis and inflammation**. Atopic, contact and endogenous (non-atopic) eczema can all produce changes in the nails (Figure 24).

Diagnosis

Most nail changes arising with eczema will do so in the presence of periungual inflammation. This is not always the case, as endogenous eczema may be manifested at sites distant to the nails, with pitting in the nails. A severe episode of local or generalised eczema may leave Beau's lines (transverse grooves) in all nails.

Periungual eczema may combine with nail pits, transverse ridging, subungual hyperkeratosis and discoloration. The

Figure 24a
Atopic eczema with normal nail folds.

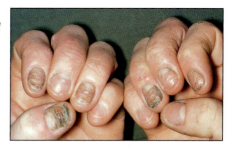

Figure 24b
Acute periungual eczema due to contact sensitivity to garlic.

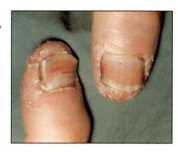

Figure 24c
Chronic irritant eczema. The dominant digits suffer most.

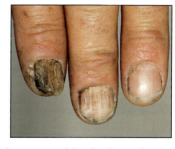

periungual involvement can be caused by both endogenous and contact eczemas: the latter includes irritant and allergic eczemas, which are most commonly found on the thumb, index and middle fingers of the dominant hand.

Distinguishing the form of eczema responsible for the nail lesions depends upon the pattern of eczema elsewhere on the body and a thorough medical, personal and occupational history. Members of certain professions are dogged by hand eczemas, particularly hairdressers and mechanics. Both of these suffer allergic and irritant contact eczemas, which often combine with an endogenous component.

Subungual hyperkeratosis is viewed as a pattern of nail-associated eczema which may merit patch testing to exclude an allergic cause. A clue as to the significance of local factors may be gained by examination of the feet. If they also are involved a contact sensitivity is less likely to be the cause, unless cosmetics are used on both hands and feet, or the hands are in contact with shoe materials. Availability of routine patch testing for hand and foot eczemas will depend upon local dermatology department facilities.

Treatment

The treatment of nail eczema involves the removal of exacerbating factors and the application of emollients (four times a day) and topical steroids (once or twice a day) to periungual skin.

Prognosis

Mild pitting with distant endogenous eczema is likely to be chronic. Palmoplantar hyperkeratotic eczemas and pompholyx have a fluctuating course which may show prolonged remissions, and the nail changes alter correspondingly. If a precipitating cause can be identified the prognosis is generally good.

Trauma and weathering

Definition

Acute mechanical and chemical trauma may leave damaged nails. However, the most common form of injury is chronic, inflicted by repetitive microtrauma or repeated immersions in minimally damaging substances.

Diagnosis of acute trauma
Haematoma
The most significant subungual sign in acute trauma is haematoma, which must be distinguished from malignant melanoma (Figure 25). The history of precipitating trauma is not always sufficient to be confident of the distinction. Features of haematoma to look for are:

- The pigmentation must be growing out with time; a firm transverse scratch at the proximal edge of the pigment will give a reference point. There should be no pigment developing proximal to this line during the assessment period.

Without these features, a biopsy may be necessary.

Chemical trauma
This is usually associated with sufficient history and soft tissue damage to give the diagnosis: a neutralising substance may assist.

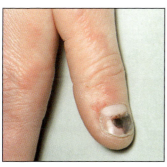

Figure 25a
Haematoma away from the proximal nail fold.

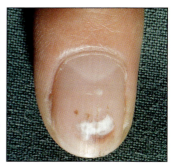

Figure 25b
Haematoma associated with traumatic transverse leuconychia.

Diagnosis of chronic trauma

Biting and picking

These are the most common forms of nail microtrauma (Figure 26). Onychotillomania is the extreme form, where the entire nail may be lost, with scarring and regrowth of any minor lateral spurs.

Median dystrophy

Another form of dystrophy probably results from minor repeated self-inflicted damage causing pressure at the base of the nail. This can arise from the common tic of pushing back the cuticle of the thumb with the index finger.

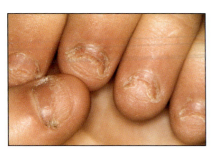

Figure 26a
Normal nail biting.

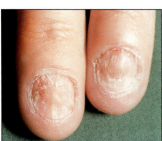

Figure 26b
Onychotillomania.

Terminal trauma

This involves recurrent minor shocks to the distal end of the nail. The cause may be **occupational** in the hands, where manual work often leads to splinter haemorrhages in the nail bed of the fingers of the dominant hand. In the

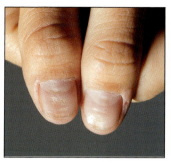

Figure 27a
Median dystrophy.
Habit-induced dystrophy.

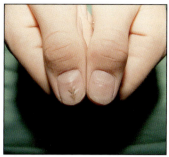

Figure 27b
Median dystrophy.
Idiopathic canaliform dystrophy.

feet terminal trauma occurs in athletes or wearers of high heels. Multiple transverse ridges are seen, most marked distally and most common in the great toe.

Athletes, particularly footballers and long-distance runners, commonly lose one or more toenails in a season. Over years, this may result in considerable permanent nail dystrophy with thickening and onycholysis.

Chronic chemical trauma
Water and/or detergent are the usual causes of this condition, which is most evident in the periungual tissues and can precipitate a paronychia. The patina of the nail may be sufficiently diminished to allow splits and cracks to develop in the distal edge.

Treatment
Treatment is always removal of the cause. It is important to remove all the offending chemicals by thorough cleansing, in order to avoid concentration of the substance beneath the distal nail margin where it may cause painful onycholysis.

Lacerating trauma near the nail matrix may require the attention of a dermatologist or hand surgeon in order to avoid a scarring dystrophy.

In nervous tics occlusion with a durable dressing, such as Granuflex®, can help. Even simple tape may suffice. In instances where the nail patina is lost, the application of nail hardeners or emollient to the nail itself may be useful.

Non-melanoma tumours

Non-melanoma tumours include the following.

Warts (see periungual and subungual warts)

Glomus tumours

Myxoid cysts

Fibromas

Subungual corns

Subungual exostoses

Bowen's disease

Invasive squamous cell carcinoma.

Glomus tumours

The tumours usually occur in 30- to 50-year-olds, and 75% present in the fingernail unit (Figure 28). When they do so they are only a few millimetres in diameter, and usually give a **substantial amount of pain** on pressure and changes in temperature. If the nail bed is involved without impingement on the matrix there may be very little to see, or just a longitudinal pink line through the nail. When the matrix is involved there is a secondary longitudinal nail dystrophy or split, which may run the entire length of the nail or may form a nick at the distal end of a groove. X-ray will sometimes show a small change in the underlying bone attributable to pressure effects. Magnetic resonance imaging gives characteristic findings. Excision of the tumour is necessary.

Figure 28
Glomus tumour.

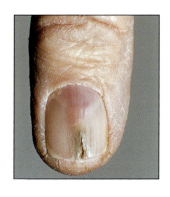

Myxoid cysts

These usually occur around the proximal nail fold and are more common in the hands than the feet (Figure 29). The cyst represents a ganglion of the distal interphalangeal joint; transillumination demonstrates a cystic quality. The tumour is usually painless but expansion may cause discomfort, relieved by incision and drainage. Pressure on the matrix can cause a longitudinal depression in the nail. The overlying proximal nail fold may become verrucous or ulcerated. The adjacent interphalangeal joint often has osteoarthritis and Heberden's nodes. Treatment requires experience: methods include plastic surgery, cryosurgery, or the cautious injection of 1% sodium tetradecyl sulphate,

Figure 29
Myxoid cyst.

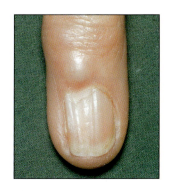

0.1 ml once a month for 3 months, after evacuation of the mucoid content. Therapy is less effective on the toes than on the fingers.

Fibromas

These may occur in the presence or absence of tuberous sclerosis (Koenen tumours) (Figure 30). They are benign dermal tumours usually seen extending from beneath the proximal or lateral nail fold onto the dorsal aspect of the nail plate. If a fibroma is solely ventral to the nail plate it may appear as a longitudinal subungual red line, with minimal symptoms. The smooth, firm morphology, emerging at the free edge or lying on the nail plate, is characteristic. A variant resembles a garlic clove, with a bulb and a small pedicle, being many small tumours compressed into one. Fibromas can be removed surgically, but it is usually necessary to reflect the nail fold to ensure extirpation of the source of the lesion.

Subungual corns

Any prolonged pressure on the nail plate, particularly from footwear or previously deformed nails, can cause these lesions (Figure 31). A subungual corn arises under the nail plate itself, typically along the distal or lateral margins of

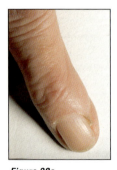

Figure 30a
Periungual fibromas.

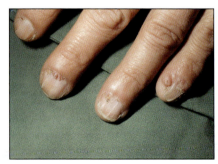

Figure 30b
Koenen tumour.

Figure 31
Subungual corn: the nail plate has been cut back to expose the lesion.

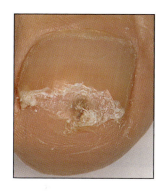

the toenails. Through the nail plate the corn usually appears yellow-brown in colour; direct pressure gives rise to pain. As the lesion develops, onycholysis may be observed in the affected toenail. Resection of the nail followed by simple debridement of the corn can give immediate relief. Attention to the cause is required if recurrence is to be avoided.

Subungual exostoses

These painful tumours usually occur in the great toe or thumb of a young adult (Figure 32). They arise beneath the distal nail and cause it to lift. The exostosis is revealed by X-ray; a lateral may be more helpful than a plane view.

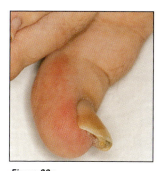

Figure 32a
Subungual exostosis.

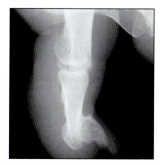

Figure 32b
X-ray of subungual exostosis.

Treatment is removal by the orthopaedic, podiatric or dermatological surgeon. In the elderly, hyperostosis may contribute to pincer nail formation, especially in the great toe.

Bowen's disease and squamous cell carcinoma

Both of these can occur around the nail unit and exist many years before the diagnosis is made (Figure 33). They may be eczematous, warty, weeping or may resemble a paronychia: all cues to delay a diagnostic biopsy. When faced with an atypical lesion that does not improve after more than 6 months of appropriate treatment, a biopsy should always be performed. Excision is the most common definitive treatment, possibly by micrographic surgery (Mohs) available through dermatological surgeons.

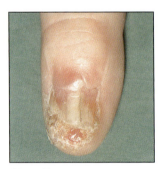

Figure 33a
Bowen's disease.

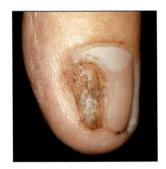

Figure 33b
Invasive squamous cell carcinoma.

Brittle nails

Definition

In this condition the nails are easily damaged. The manner of the trauma and its effects are various, with the most common results being tears, splits and fractures

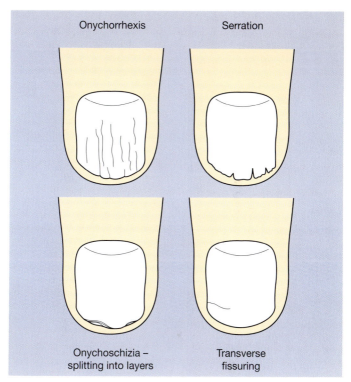

Figure 34
Four patterns of damage in brittle nails

(Figure 34). Abnormally brittle nails demonstrate one or more forms of damage at the free edge, as illustrated in Figure 35.

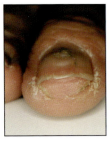

Figure 35a
Chemical periungual/nail damage in a cement worker.

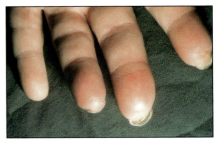

Figure 35b
Nails in Raynaud's disease/systemic sclerosis.

Causes

The most common causes are non-specific: old age and frequent immersion of the hands in water with subsequent drying. Other causes are as follows.

Local	**Trauma**
	Psoriasis
	Onychomycosis
	Chemicals: alkalis, detergents, oils, solvents
	Lichen planus
General	**Chronic arthropathy**
	Iron deficiency
	Peripheral vascular disease
	Cachexia
	Hemiplegia
	Vitamin A, B_6 or C deficiency

Treatment

The cause should be removed if possible. Hands need protection from wetting (barrier creams are not helpful). Emollient applied twice daily to a hydrated nail can help to maintain moisture and diminish brittleness. This should also be done after each immersion, to reduce the repeated drying-out that makes the nails brittle. Base coat, nail polish and top coat may act both to splint the nail and to retain moisture.

Ingrowing nails – onychocryptosis

Definition

We describe the condition as seen in adults and adolescents. In the most common form the great toe is affected (Figure 36). **The nail grows into the lateral nail fold, causing trauma, inflammation and secondary infection**. Hypergranulation tissue may protrude from the sulcus. Four main categories are recognised in the adult, as follows.

Figure 36
Onychocryptosis following conservative removal of the offending nail spicule. The resected spike of nail can be seen just below on the great toe.

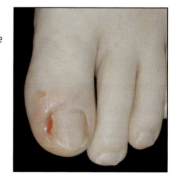

Subcutaneous ingrowing nail

This often appears as a result of improper trimming of the nail (Figure 37). A sharp spicule of nail at the edge grows into the soft tissue of the lateral nail fold.

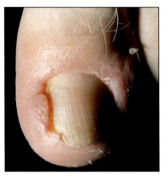

Figure 37
Badly clipped nail invading lateral nail fold.

Hypertrophy of the lateral nail fold

Longstanding trauma between the nail and lateral nail fold may result in the overgrowth of the soft tissues (Figure 38). This tissue forms a lip that overrides the nail.

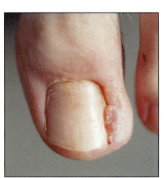

Figure 38
Hypertrophy of the lateral nail fold with embedded nail.

Pincer or involuted nail

Pincer or involuted nail is defined as an over-curvature of the lateral nail edges towards the nail bed (Figure 39). The excess curvature is seen most commonly in the great toe, where it may lead to chronic pain and inflammation as the subungual tissues are compressed.

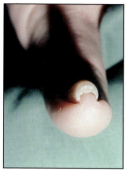 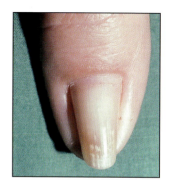

Figure 39
Pincer nail, embedding.

Distal nail embedding

If the great toenail is lost for any reason, it may grow into, rather than over, the distal nail bed as it regenerates (Figure 40).

Figure 40
Distal embedding of nail with regrowth after nail loss.

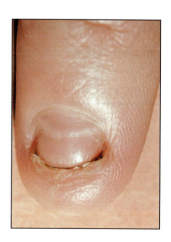

Causes

Ingrowing nails are usually acquired and attributed to poorly fitting shoes, sport, aggressive manicure, nail-biting or other trauma. There is a basic disproportion between the nail and lateral nail fold, resulting in damage to the latter. In pincer nail the most frequent cause is pressure on the nail plate from footwear or deformed digits, although when many nails are affected a family history may exist. Occasionally, isolated cases may result from an underlying exostosis.

General treatments

Acute ingrowing toenails

If infection is suspected a swab should be taken and appropriate antibiotics given. Initial episodes may be treated by skilled conservative resection and retrieval of the offending nail spike, followed by daily hypertonic saline footbaths until resolution occurs. Patients should also be advised on cutting nails straight across avoiding the nail corners. Footwear should be assessed.

Chronic ingrowing toenails

If conservative treatment fails or the condition is recurrent, nail surgery should be considered. As much as possible of the nail plate should be preserved. There is seldom need to remove the entire nail. The treatment of choice is partial nail avulsion, i.e. removal of the lateral quarter of the nail including the associated matrix.

The procedure is as follows.

- Anaesthesia of the toe is achieved through a ring block of the digit.

- A tourniquet is applied.

- The lateral quarter of the nail is lifted from the nail bed and split using a nail chisel or Thwaites nippers.

- Using locking forceps, the nail wedge is medially rotated until it separates completely.

- The area is cleared of debris.

- A solution of phenol is applied for 3 minutes.

- The area is dried and a dressing is applied.

- Resolution usually occurs in 2 to 3 weeks, but may take up to 6 weeks.

When wound healing may be a problem, other excisional techniques should be considered.

Cryosurgery of the exuberant lateral nail fold can be successful.

Particular treatments

Treatment of **hypertrophy of the lateral nail fold** is by an elliptical excision of soft tissue from beneath the affected area, allowing it to drop down out of the path of nail growth. In addition, the nail may be narrowed by phenolisation of the lateral horn of the matrix.

In **pincer nails**, conservative nail care may give symptomatic relief. The involuted nail edges are regularly cut back and filed smooth to relieve pressure on the nail bed. Footwear should also be checked for fit over the affected digits. In more severe cases, pincer nails may predispose to subungual corns (see non-melanoma tumours) and painful inflammation of the digit. In such cases nail surgery is indicated. Before surgery is undertaken it is advisable to inspect a lateral X-ray of the toe, to rule out subungual exostosis as a cause of the problem.

When there is distal nail embedding, therapy may involve surgery to drop the level of the nail bed and so allow unrestricted growth of the nail

Index